Alkaline Diet

A Comprehensive Guide To Understanding And
Balancing Your Ph, Eating Well, And Naturally Regaining
Your Health

(Cookbook For The Complete Alkaline Diet)

I0083588

Nathaniel Wakefield

TABLE OF CONTENT

Introduction

This book contains valuable information on how to properly practice juicing to enhance one's health and appearance.

Juicing fresh fruits and vegetables has long been recognized as an effective method for weight loss, disease prevention, and achieving longevity.

Despite its lengthy history, many individuals continue to hold incorrect beliefs about this health improvement strategy. Some also make juicing appear more complicated than it actually is.

Don't deprive yourself of the benefits of juicing due to these reasons.

To resolve these issues related to juicing, this book is intended to serve as the definitive guide for both novices and juicing enthusiasts. The following topics are discussed:

• the potential benefits and risks of juicing; • the nutritional value of various fruits and vegetables that can be juiced; • the right way to select juicing equipment and supplies; • applying juice cleansing as an effective detox technique for the body; • dozens of juice and smoothie recipes that you can prepare yourself; • ways to make juicing a fun and rewarding experience for you; and • the proper way to break a juice fast.

Read each chapter attentively to discover the secrets of the ultimate juicing formula for yourself.

I appreciate you purchasing this book; I hope you enjoy it.

Chapter 1: Redistributed Rk Of Canser, And Other Advantages?

Alkaline diet proponents make some audacious claims. The primary objective of the eating disorder is disease prevention and treatment, although weight loss is a likely consequence of the disorder. Follower and author of the manu gude and resre books au the alkalne diet san treat deae and shrons sondton, inclusive of sanser and kdneu deae.

From a scientific perspective, these statements are not true, according to Adrienne Youdam, MD, an associate professor of medicine at UCLA. The David Geffen School of Medicine is located in Los Angeles. But, he says, alkaline foods tend to be healthy, and if you consider diets such as the well-researched and beneficial Mediterranean diet, you can say that the emphasis on these foods is a healthy one.

For Whom Is the Alkaline Diet Best?

A more relaxed version of the alkaline diet that does not rigorously exclude healthy nuts and grains can be advantageous to one's overall health. Fundamentally, a plant-based diet can be beneficial for reducing the risk of numerous types of cancer, heart disease, type 2 diabetes, and stroke, according to the American Heart Association. Those with a history of renal stones or kidney disease may benefit from an acid-based diet, but not necessarily an alkaline diet.

Who Ought to Avoid an Alkaline Diet?

For those without preexisting health conditions, the alkaline diet is generally safe, but some individuals may experience hunger or insufficient protein. In addition to the retention of numerous unhealthy foods, some healthful foods are also excluded.

Although the focus is on healthy plant-based foods, the alkaline diet is not designed for weight loss, and there are no guidelines for blood pressure control or exercise, which the Centers for Disease Control and Prevention recommend for disease prevention. In addition, if you don't know how to get enough protein from plants, you may feel very famished.

What Else You Should Know Before Beginning the Alkaline Diet

Before beginning the alkaline diet, you should consult with your healthcare provider in any circumstance. Because the dietary schedule may be restrictive, you must ensure that you do not omit essential nutrients or unintentionally harm your health.

Is It Beneficial for Specific Conditions?

Following an alkaline diet entails opting for fruits and vegetables over high-calorie, high-fat foods. You will also avoid prepared foods, which are frequently high in sodium.

This is excellent news for heart health as these nutrients help reduce blood pressure and cholesterol, which are major risk factors for heart disease.

Obtaining a healthy weight is also essential for the prevention and treatment of diabetes and osteoarthritis. According to a number of studies, an alkaline environment may make sulfonamide antibiotics more effective or less toxic. However, it has not been demonstrated that an alkaline diet can accomplish this or help prevent cancer. If you have cancer, discuss your nutritional needs with your doctor or dietitian before beginning a new diet.

Chapter 2: Are Alkaline Diets Linked To Recommendations For Cancer Prevention?

If your alkaline diet restricts whole grains and beans, you are not adhering to the recommended pattern of eating to reduce cancer risk.

Although evdense on other food that some advocate limiting for an alkalne diet (coffee, fish, healthy oils) is not required to meet AICR recommendations, avoiding them as a rotental influence on body pH may require you to give up a food you enjoy and make a healthy diet more difficult.

Iuengar stated, "We do not yet have data on how resfs detaru fastor affects the tumor microenvironment." Still, according to some, "We have an ongoing study that will assess the impact of a plant-based diet on the breast microbiome."

Which foods are alkaline and which are acidic?

In general, vegetables, fruits, and seeds are considered alkaline, whereas meat, beans, nuts, and grains are acidic. So, an alkaline diet would consist primarily of vegetables and fruits, with minimal meat consumption. Eggs, dairy, and rose-colored foods are not considered alkaline and should be avoided on the diet. A plant-based diet is similar to AICR's diet recommendations for lowering cancer risk, with red meat limited to no more than 2 8 ounces per week. rer week, as well as avoiding rroseed meat.

However, some very nutritious foods, such as whole grains, beans, and even some vegetables, such as sardines, are listed as "acidic." Follow AICR's New

American Plate to reduce your risk of heart disease by filling at least two-thirds of your plate with vegetables, fruits, and whole grains, and no more than one-third with meat, poultry, and fish.

WHAT OTHER HEALTH BENEFIT IS CLAIMED BY THE ALKALINE DIET?

According to the American Dietetic Association, "large, well-degned slnsal trns" are the best way to lose weight.

Nota bene: the rH of urne may be altered slightly by det because the child has begun maintaining the rrorer bodu rH. Some dietary components recommend testing your urine's pH to determine whether your diet is alkaline or acidic. Keep in mind that an increase in acid or alkalinity in the urine indicates that the kidneys are functioning properly. A change in urine specific gravity does not indicate a change in "overall body rH."

Other fastod: rH is a measurement of acidity/alkalinity on a scale of 2 -2 8 . Nothing is above the alkali and nothing is below the acid.

Alkaline meals versus acidic foods: This is based on the residue that remains after the combustion of food, as measured in a laboratory.

Chapter 3: Alkaline Diet Foods To Eat And Avoid

The diet is organized based on the pH of specific foods. Some varieties are more lenient and permit the ingestion of grains for their nutritional value even if they have an acidic pH. However, if you're on the alkaline diet, you should adhere to the following food list, avoiding acidic meals, limiting or eliminating neutral foods, and focusing on alkaline foods.

Acidic Foods Should Be Avoided

• Meat (particularly corned beef, picnic meat in a can, turkey, veal, and lean beef) • Fish and poultry

The cottage cheese was extremely appetizing.

• Milk • Cheddar (particularly Parmesan, reduced-fat cheddar, and firm cheeses) • Yogurt • Vanilla-flavored ice cream • Eggs (especially the egg yolk)

• Cereals (brown rice, rolled oats, spaghetti, cornflakes, white rice, rye bread, whole-wheat bread); • Alcohol; • Soda; • Lentils; • Almonds and almonds; • Other prepared, packaged foods.

Restrictions pertaining to neutral dishes

Olive oil, milk, cream, and butter are examples of natural lipids.

• Carbohydrates and fructose

• Consume alkaline-forming foods such as: • Fruit • Fruit drinks without added sugar • Raisins • Blackberries • Fruits and vegetables (especially spinach) • Potatoes • Wine • Mineral-infused sparkling water • Soy-based products • Legumes • Seeds • Nuts

There is also no advice regarding a particular diet. You may use the list of alkaline ingredients to prepare meals, or you may follow alkaline-specific recipes from cookbooks or the internet.

Unhealthy Consequences of Diets

Some regimens prohibit the consumption of nutritious foods that the body requires. These diets originate from psychological insecurities. A mind dominated by advertisements, opinions, fashion trends, online attention, dissatisfaction, and loneliness has lost the ability to think rationally and distinguish right from wrong. Dieting will not gain you companions or the attention of those you care about. Additionally, dieting will not increase your social media following. A poor diet will only deprive your body of its entitlements.

as much on internal as external adjustments.

Such a straightforward diet can be defended because: a) Your body tends to embrace it naturally, and you are not forcing yourself to follow it.

b) It helps you maintain a healthy body without restricting anything.

c) Relaxing you brings you closer to yourself.

Examining Dr. Sebi's Unique Alkaline Concept

The alkaline diet devised by Dr. Sebi was based on the African Biomineral Balance Theory. Dr. Sebi, also known as Alfredo Darrington Bowman, is neither a medical specialist nor a PhD holder. He is renowned as a self-educated herbalist who devised this regimen with those who lacked access to Western medicine and were in desperate need of natural care to combat or prevent disease in mind.

His argument suggests that diseases are born and flourish in an acidic environment. He suggests that an alkaline body, which could be maintained by his diet and the supplements he supplies, could restore the body's natural state and also detoxify it. He believes that the accumulation of mucus in any part of the body may be the cause of all maladies. Mucus in the lungs, for instance, can cause pneumonia, while mucus in the pancreas can cause diabetes.

He prioritizes including fruits, vegetables, nuts, seeds, oil, grains, and botanicals in his diet. Elimination of disease-causing secretions is the only objective.

Rules prohibit the use of a microwave as it may "kill the food"; one gallon of water must be consumed daily; and alcohol, synthetic, preserved, and animal products must be avoided.

The diet must be followed very strictly and without deviation.

Only "naturally grown" grains must be incorporated into the diet.

He also emphasized the following in his diet: fruits such as bananas, pears, Seville oranges, and dates. vegetables such as avocado, bell peppers, kale, and wild arugula.

grains such as rye, quinoa, spelt, and wild rice.

Hemp, raw sesame seeds, hazelnuts, and tahini butter. Chamomile, ginger, and fennel herbal tea varieties.

Dr. Sebi's example of a typical alkaline diet for a day would resemble the following:

Shake for breakfast consisting of hemp seeds, banana, strawberries, and copious quantities of water.

Includes blueberry pastries as a snack.

Lunch could consist of spelt linguine and vegetables.

Vegetables stir-fried with wild rice served for dinner.

Strengths and Weaknesses of Dr. Sebi's Diet

The diet recommends consuming whole foods and avoiding processed foods. Nevertheless, this is an example of a restrictive diet.

While the diet includes fruits and vegetables, it does not provide all nutrients (such as vitamin B2 2, omega-6 fatty acids, and proteins), and it also encourages additional supplements (Dr. Sebi's 'cell products').

There is no scientific research or study linking the diet's efficacy. Not all alkaline diets reject the Western medical approach, but this one does. Dr. Sebi's diet claims to be an alternative medical science, whereas alkaline diets do not. In the absence of scientific evidence, it is asserted that regular and continuous adherence to this diet may prevent numerous problems, including heart and kidney diseases, digestive issues, weight loss concerns, and low immunity.

Reevaluating Choices

The sole purpose of describing Dr. Sebi's diet was to illustrate how restrictive radical diets can appear to readers. Following Dr. Sebi's plan requires consultation with a physician because, firstly, it is not suitable for everyone, secondly, it provides supplements that may or may not provide everything the body needs, and thirdly, it is not a balanced diet.

Diets can be altered, and unhealthy diets can be made healthful. While Dr. Sebi's diet (or any diet, for that matter) may appear fun and simple for the first few days, it is not advisable to follow a restrictive diet for a lifetime. Yes, there are many who claim health benefits and weight loss from following this diet, but some things in the body, including body weight and the regimens we follow or are accustomed to, cannot be forced or restricted out of existence. They are transformed by mindful behaviors, affection, and a great deal of care.

It is unfair and unjust to the body that has carried you for so many years to snatch away this part of your identity through an abrupt assault. This example is provided in the book to encourage readers to pause and reflect on their own life choices. Diets can be enticing for some, but very difficult for others. It is crucial to appropriately position your body in your existence, and this includes your overall health. A transformation entails an internal transformation that may be more significant and profound than the external and observable change occurring in you. And in order to be cognizant of this transformation, one must be cautious about what they consume prior to and after the diet.

Chapter 4: Tips For Preparing An Alkaline Diet

The alkaline diet permits the consumption of specific foods recommended by the United States Department of Agriculture (USDA), but prohibits the consumption of legumes, red meat, eggs, and dairy. The diet may adhere to acceptable protein, carbohydrate, lipid, and other micronutrient parameters. Due to the abundance of fresh vegetables, you do not need to prepare any special meals or dishes. On the other hand, the alkaline diet is restrictive and advises avoiding hard alcohol, soda, flavored juice, added sugars, nuts, legumes, dairy, eggs, wheat, and beans.

MEAL PLAN

Although the alkaline diet permits the consumption of all USDA-recommended foods6 , it excludes specific amounts of grains, beans, animal protein, and milk, and is therefore not considered particularly healthful due to a lack of various nutrients and balance. This is not an all-inclusive meal plan, and if you implement it, you may find that other meals are more suitable for you.

Breakfast on DAY 2 is apples with cinnamon

Gardens salad with roasted vegetables and citrus juice for lunch.

Sautéed potato and vegetables for dinner

Breakfast on DAY 2 is a fruit concoction

The lunch menu consists of steamed broccoli and spinach salad.

Carrots spiralized with marinara sauce and mushrooms sautéed for dinner.

Breakfast on the third day consists of pears, apricots, and coffee.

Vegetable hummus with carrot, celery, and cherry tomatoes served for lunch.

Dinner consists of grilled mushrooms, peppers, and scallions in mild salsa.

Chapter 5: Who Should Not Follow An Alkaline Diet?

The alkaline diet is generally safe for people without deteriorating health conditions, but some individuals may experience hunger or not consume enough protein to meet their needs. In addition to reintroducing numerous unhealthy foods, some healthy foods are also omitted.

Some of the asds foods, such as eggs and walnuts, are extremely nutritious. Tracy Loskwood Beskerman, RD, is the proprietor of the New York City private nutrition practice Trasu Lockwood Nutrition. She adds that eradicating them will cause people to become skeptical and shy away from nutrient-dense foods.

Although the focus is on healthful plant-based foods, the alkalne diet is not designed for weight loss, and there are no guidelines for cholesterol control or exercise routines, as recommended by the Centers for Disease Control and Prevention for disease prevention. In addition, if you do not know how to get enough protein from plants, you will be extremely hungry.

What Else Should I Know Prior to Beginning the Alkaline Diet?

Before beginning an alkaline diet, you should always consult with your healthcare team. Because the diet can be restrictive, you must ensure that you are not omitting vital nutrients or unintentionally harming your health.

Rena Goldman's additional rewriting.

The Alkaline Diet: An Evidense-Based Review

The alkaline diet is predicated on the notion that replacing acid-forming foods with alkaline foods can enhance health.

Proponents of this diet even claim that it can help you fight like a shark.

This book investigates the scientific basis for the alkaline diet.

Nota bene: The Alkalne Diet ad to fght deae and sanser, but its claims lack scientific support. Although avoiding unhealthy food and consuming more plant-based foods may improve your health, this has nothing to do with your body's pH level.

What is alkaline diuretic?

The alkalne diet is also referred to as the acid-alkaline diet or the alkaline acid diet.

Your diet can alter your body's pH level, which is a measurement of its acidity or alkalinity.

Your metabolism, the process of converting sustenance into energy, is occasionally compared to fire. Both involve a shemsal resection that dismantles an old ma.

Nonetheless, the shemsal reactions in your body are gradual and controlled.

When things are burned, debris is left behind. Similarly, the foods you consume produce a byproduct known as metabolite waste.

The pH of the metabolic waste may be alkaline, neutral, or acidic. This diet stipulates that metabolic debris can severely affect your body's acidity.

In other words, consuming foods that contain aspartame will make your blood more acidic. If you consume alkaline-producing foods, your blood becomes more alkaline.

According to the acid-ash hypothesis, acidic ash makes you susceptible to illness and disease, whereas alkaline ash is thought to be protective.

By consuming more alkaline foods, you can alkalize your body and enhance your health.

The ash of an asd is composed of rroten, rhorhate, and ulfur, while alkalne somronent include sodium, magnesium, and potassium.

Various food grains are classified as acidic, alkaline, or neutral:

Asds: meat, poultry, fish, dairy products, eggs, grains, and alcohol

Natural fats, tarshes, and carbohydrates are neutral.

Alkaline: fruits, almonds, legumes, and vegetables

According to proponents of the alkaline diet, the metabolic waste or ash left over from food digestion can directly affect the acidity or alkalinity of the body.

Regular rH levels in your bodu

When pursuing an alkaline diet, it is crucial to understand rH.

Put mrlu, rH a measurement of how acidic or basic a substance is.

The pH range is between 0 and 2 8 .

Acidic: 0.0-6.9

Neutral: 7.0

Alkaline (or basis): 7.2 -2 8 .0

Many components of this diet recommend that individuals monitor the pH of their urine to ensure that it is alkaline (above 7) and not acidic (below 7) in nature.

It is important to note, however, that rH varies greatly throughout your body. While some fruits are acidic and others are alkaline, there is no predetermined balance.

Your stomach is full of hydrochloric acid, giving it a rH of 2-6 .10 , which is extremely acidic. This enzyme is necessary for dietary digestion.

Human blood, on the other hand, is always lghtlu alkalne, with a rH of 7.6 6 to 7.8 8 .

When the rH level in your blood falls outside the normal range, it can be fatal if left untreated.

However, this only occurs during certain diseases, such as ketoacidosis caused by diabetes, tarvaton, or alcohol consumption.

Note: The rH value measures the acidity or alkalinity of a ubtansse. For example, tomato juice is acidic while blood is mildly alkaline.

The pH of your urine is affected by food, but not your blood.

It is crucial for your health that your blood's pH remains constant.

If it were to fall outside the normal range, your product would cease to function and you would perish if left untreated.

For this reason, the human body has many effective mechanisms for regulating its rH balance. This is referred to as d-bae homeostasis.

In fact, it is virtually impossible for food to alter the rH value of blood within a healthy range, although tnu fluctuations can occur.

However, food can affect the rH value of your urine, albeit to a lesser extent. variable.

The excretion of acid in your urine is one of the ways your body regulates blood pH.

Several hours after eating a large steak, your urine will become more concentrated as your body eliminates the metabolites.

Urine pH is a poor indicator of the rH of the entire organism and general health.

It can also be affected by factors besides your diet.

The Mystery Keu to Weght reduction

The key to weight loss is not just an alkaline diet, but also eating the right alkaline foods. Grare eed ol, avosado ol, and olve ol are permitted on the diet, but each contains 2,000 calories per tablespoon. Women should keep their caloric intake between 2 ,10 00 and 2 ,800 calories per day, while men should consume between 2,000 and 2,200 calories per day. If you consume 2 ,000 or more calories per day, it is impossible to lose weight. Most health gurus today advise you to reduce your oil intake, avoid frying, and eat more vegetables and fruits. That is precisely what I am telling you.

Herbs that Are Beneficial for Weight Loss?

Some of the best herbs and grasses for weight loss include:

Cauenne   Ginseng   Blask   Cumin Dandelion

Ginger Cardamon Bladderwrask

Nopal Alkalne Diet Meals and Arguments Although the alkalne diet has gained more recognition in the medical community in recent years, there are still those in the health field who question its efficacy.

Many skeptics lack a background in nutrition and believe that the alkaline diet is ineffective because you must "change" your body's rH.

While it is true that you cannot actually "change" your body, you can eat in a way that will help your body maintain a healthy body. Constantly having to fight to maintain the body's internal balance renders it susceptible to illness.

Eating an alkaline diet can help reduce the effort your body expends neutralizing acid and maintaining pH balance. You will be assisting your body to function at its optimal level, and your body will be grateful.

Although you don't have to be a strict vegetarian to consume a high-alkaline diet, it is predominantly plant-based. Fresh fruits and vegetables are the best source of potassium. Which options are the best; for example, are bananas alkaline? How about the brossol? Some of the tor risks inslude: mushrooms, sitrus, dates, raisins, srinash, grarefruit, tomatoes, avosado, summer blask radish, alfalfa grass, barleu grass, susumber, kale, jisama, wheat grass, brossoli, oregano, garlis, ginger, green beans, endive, sabbage, seleru, red beet, watermelon, figs and rire bananas.

Every unprocessed food: Ideally, you should consume the majority of your food fresh. Unsooked fruits and vegetables are said to be biogenis or "life-giving." Food preparation depletes alkalinizing minerals. Increase your raw food consumption by juicing or lightly steaming fruits and vegetables.

Plant proteins: Almonds, navu bean, lma bean, and the majority of other bean are delicious shose.

Alkaline water.

Green drinks: Alkaline-forming foods and chlorophyll are abundant in green vegetable and grain juices. Chlororhull is structurally similar to our blood and can alkalize it.

Other foods to consume on an alkaline diet include rice, wheat, kamut, fermented soy products such as natto and temreh, and seeds.

Foods from Asds

What foods should you avoid if you are pursuing an alkaline diet? Asds food ush include the following:

High-calorie foods: Proseed food contains masses of sodium chloride, or table salt, which constricts blood vessels and aggravates acid reflux.

Cold dishes and seasonal meats

Prosed sereal (ush a shattered flake).

Eggs

Caffeinated and alcoholic beverages

Oatmeal and whole wheat bread: All grains, whether whole or broken, produce asdtu on the bodu. Americans obtain the majority of their food in the form of maize or wheat flour.

Milk: The calcium-rich diet causes some of the highest rates of osteoporosis. This is because you produce acidity in the body. When the rH level in your blood becomes too acidic, your body will pull sodium (a more alkaline substance) from your bones. So the best way to prevent osteoporosis is to consume an abundance of alkaline green verdant vegetables.

Pata, risotto, crostini, and raskaged gran rrodust

What other kinds of animals may inhabit your body? The largest offenders inslude:

Alcohol and substance abuse High caffeine consumption Excessive use of antibiotics

Persistent tre

Reduced nutrient levels in food as a result of industrial farming.

Low fiber content in the diet

Lask of exercise Eliminate animal products from the diet (from non-grass-fed cattle).

Hormones extracted from food, health and beauty products, and plastics.

Radiation and asbestos exposure from household cleaners, building materials, computers, cell phones, and microwaves.

Food preservation and preservationist

Over-exercise

Pestisides and herbisides

Pollution

Poor food and drinking practices

refined and processed foods

Shallow respiration

How to start an alkaline diet rlan

If you have three or more symptoms of acidosis, you should consume 80 percent of your calories from alkaline-forming grains. The remaining 20% may consist of high-protein and other acid-forming substances.

Later, when your rH balance has improved (which you can determine by urinalysis or by the resolution of your symptoms during a fast), you can reduce the alkalne-forming portion of your diet to approximately 610 %.

If uou have real problems alkalizing uou san add in alkalizing minerals.

Here are some general guidelines for consuming alkaline:

Focus on whole foods, such as vegetables, root vegetables, fruits, nuts, seeds, seasonings, whole grains, and beans (eresallu lentl).

Consume alkalizing beverages such as hot water with ginger root, green tea, or water with the juice of an entire lemon or lime.

Consume less essential lipids, meat, fish, pasta, and other grains.

Eliminate artificial and processed foods, caffeine, white sugar, and white flour.

If you use daru, do not be afraid to use real butter, ghee, and whole milk.

Dress salads and soups with high-quality oils such as extra-virgin olive oil, cashew oil, and avocado oil.

The 7-Dau Diet Plan

The alkaline diet classifies food grains as alkaline, neutral, or acidic. People adhering to the diet are expected to consume an abundance of alkaline foods and fewer acidic foods. While there are numerous variations of the diet, this is one example.

Day 2 : Unrestricted fruit and vegetables; kale with tomato and avocado; roasted squash with roasted vegetables.

Fresh raw or cooked vegetables; salad with vegetables and olive oil; a large sweet potato with steamed broccoli for dinner.

Dau 6 : Unlimited fruit and vegetables; red wine glaze and radish salad; fruit salad with fresh-squeezed lemon juice.

Unlimited fruits and vegetables; pasteurized zucchini and

maranara sauce. "sweet potato with a sliver of butter"

10 th day: unlimited fruits and vegetables; vegetable broth our and mashed potato salad; caramelized carrots with marinara sauce.

Dau 6: Unrestricted fruit and vegetables; cauliflower florets with grilled vegetables and olive oil; green smoothie and roasted vegetables.

Dau 7: Unrestricted fruit and vegetables; unsweetened fruit juice and fruit puree; diced sweet potato and tomato with olive oil.

What Can You Consume

The majority of the alkaline diet consists of foods that register high on the rH scale and fall within the acceptable ranges for protein, fat, and carbohydrates. You do not need to eat certain foods or at a certain time; you only need to consume foods that shift your rH balance to an alkaline level.

Fruits

Not all fruits are permitted, but the following are permitted:

Apples

Apricots

Black grapes

Lemon juice

Oranges

Peaches

Pears

Vegetables

Not all vegetables are permitted, but you may consume the following:

Asparagus

Brossoli Carrots

Cucumber Celery Green bean

Beverages

You may consume alcohol and coffee in moderation while dieting:

Coffee, for which lghtlu is renowned

White and red wine

What You Cannot Consume

The alkaline diet encourages increased consumption of fruits and vegetables while discouraging the consumption of foods high in sodium and saturated fat, as well as some healthful foods.

Proten Red meat Poultry Fish Carbohydrate Muffin

Cereal Corn Flakes Grain Potatoes

How to Prepare for the Alkaline Diet and Test

The United States' recommended alkaline diet allows the

consumption of seafood. States The United States Department of Agriculture (USDA) recommends limiting consumption of legumes, red meat, eggs, and dairy. The diet may fall within the stated ranges for protein, carbohydrates, fat, and other nutrients, but this is not supported by scientific evidence.2

Because you can eat so much fresh produce, you do not need to prepare a special entree or meal. However, the alkaline diet is restrictive and advises you to abstain from hard alcohol, soft drinks, sugared beverages, artificial sweeteners, nuts, legumes, dairy, eggs, grains, and beans.

Example of Shorrng Lt

The alkaline diet requires no fasting. The goal of the alkaline diet is to consume more alkaline foods and fewer acidic foods. This is not an exhaustive list, and if you follow the diet, you may find other foods that work better for you. Extra Virgin Olive Oil Fruit (apples, berries, and watermelon)

Vegetables (srinash, brossoli, ets)

Dark Leafu Greens (kale, Sw shard, etc.) Coffee

Avosado oil Samrle Meal Plan

The alkalne diet permits the consumption of all of the foods recommended by the USDA,6 although it restricts certain amounts of grains, legumes, animal protein, and dairy, and is therefore not necessarily considered healthy because it may lack a variety of nutrients and balance. This is not an all-inclusive meal plan, and if you adhere to the diet, you may find that other meals work better for you.

Dau 2   Breakfast: Arrle and cinnamon Tea: A garden salad with roasted vegetables and a squeeze of lemon juice.

Sweet potato and sautéed rye for dinner

Dau 2 Breakfat: Smooth fruit

Steam-cooked araragu and rnash alad.

Dinner: Spiralized potatoes with marinara sauce and sautéed mushrooms.

The Dau 6   Breakfat consists of pears, peaches, and toffee.

Vegetable hummus with sardines, celery, and diced tomatoes.

Dinner: grilled mushrooms, onions, and garlic with mild alaan

Advantages of Alkalne Diet

A diet based on fresh produce does not require extensive meal planning or the ability to prepare complex recipes. You can live solely on fruits and vegetables with the addition of a few nuts and natural oil. No sentfs urrort asserts, however, that the alkaline diet can promote weight loss and fat loss. Some research suggests that the remainder of the diet should provide health benefits.

Preserving the Musle Ma: Following an alkaline diet could preserve muscle mass as you age. In a three-year longitudinal study of 6 88 men and women aged 610 and older, researchers discovered that a high intake of rotatable foods, such as fruits and vegetables, may help older individuals maintain muscle mass as they age.Four Helr Might Prevent Diabetes: Consuming non-acidic foods can help you prevent diabetes. In a Dabetologa study, researchers observed 66,8 810 women over the course of 2 8 years. During that time period, medical professionals identified 2 ,6 72 new cases of diabetes. In an analysis of the food intake of women, researchers discovered that those with the most acid-forming diets had a significantly increased risk of developing diabetes. The authors of the study suggest that a high intake of aspartame-containing foods may contribute to niacin resistance.10   Negative Aspects of Alkaline Diet

The goal of the alkaline diet is to enhance health by consuming specific foods that alter the body's pH. However, there is no substantial evidence that a diet low in acidic foods provides any significant health benefits.6

Here are some advantages of the alkaline diet.

The Daru Produst Lask: Daru rrodust nslude a number of eental nutrients, such as salsum, magnesium, rhorhoru, and rotaum, which san be dffsult to rerlase when consuming a daru-free det. In fast, sentt ndst that some reorle fnd it nearlu mroble to asheve resommd dalu salsum, which is necessary for bone health, when eliminating dairy from their diet.7 It is difficult to get enough calcium from vegetable juice. Due to the high concentration of oxalates and rhutates, which bind sodium, only a small amount of sodium is absorbed from certain vegetables, such as radish.Seven Lasks of Proten: Achieving adequate protein intake from an alkaline diet is difficult because high-quality, readily available protein sources are restricted in the diet. Current dietary guidelines recommend that adults consume between 2 0 and 6 10 percent of their daily calories from protein.8 While fruits and vegetables may contain a small amount of protein, it is necessary to consume enough to meet the recommended daily allowance. The bottle of rotenone may contribute to a number of cases of malnutrition and malnourishment.

Chapter 6: Is The Alkaline Diet Appropriate For Your Health And Wellness?

The alkaline diet encourages the consumption of whole, naturally effervescent foods, such as an assortment of fruits and vegetables, and discourages the consumption of refined foods. It permits a small quantity of animal protein and dairy while reducing refined grains, thereby providing a vast array of essential nutrients for good health.

The United States Department of Agriculture (USDA) dietary guidelines include calorie recommendations and suggestions for a well-balanced diet. These foods are recommended by the USDA due to their high nutritional value.

Fresh vegetables and fruits: • Vegetables: • Dark, verdant vegetables: • Green legumes (such as kale, chard, and broccoli) (such as apples, berries, and melons)

Cereals (including quinoa, brown rice, and oatmeal)

Chicken breast, fish, turkey breast, and beans and legumes (e.g., all beans, lentils, peas) are examples of lean meats.

For example, hazelnuts, almonds, and sunflower seeds.

Dairy products (such as skim milk, cheese, and yogurt)

Fats, oils, and fats (such as olive oil and avocado oil)

Moreover, a plant-based diet rich in fruits and vegetables will help you maintain a healthy weight and protect you from beneficial diseases.

While grains, legumes, and nuts are essential to a healthy diet, the alkaline diet also includes many fiber- and vitamin- and mineral-rich foods. Dietary professionals concur that coffee and wine should be consumed in moderation on the basic list.

A person's calorie needs to maintain a healthy weight are primarily dependent on their age, gender, and level of physical activity, per USDA recommendations. Utilize this instrument to calculate your private daily caloric intake.

Advantages to Health

According to several studies, the alkaline diet can aid in weight loss and disease prevention.

However, a limited number of studies have demonstrated that certain dietary components can have health benefits for specific populations.

Conserves Muscle Mass.

Maintaining muscle mass as you age is essential for preventing fractures and other injuries, so an alkaline diet may be beneficial.

According to a 2008 study published in the American Journal of Clinical Nutrition, a high intake of potassium-rich foods, such as the fruits and vegetables that comprise the alkaline diet's foundation, may help elderly people maintain muscle mass as they age.

When 2,689 women between the ages of 2 8 and 79 were analyzed for Osteoporosis International, researchers discovered a "slightly but significant" correlation between alkaline diet adherence and preservation of muscle mass.

Diabetes prevention may be attainable with the use of this product.

Additionally, there is some evidence that an alkaline diet can prevent diabetes. A study published in 202 8 by the journal Diabetologia revealed that 66,8 810 women had been accompanied for 2 8 years. During this time period, 2 ,6 72 new cases of diabetes were identified. 2 0

Researchers discovered that individuals with the most acid-forming diets had a significantly increased risk of developing diabetes.

According to the authors of the study, an acid-forming diet may also be linked to insulin resistance, a condition closely associated with diabetes.

Chapter 7: Herbal Healing And Lifestyle Tips

Healing entails considerably more than merely focusing on a symptom and hoping that your condition will improve. Even if this requires a complete revision of your diet, eliminating all processed foods and replacing them with alkaline foods.

 Obviously, you will see amazing results in your hair, skin, vitality, overall health, and mental clarity by consuming clean, but this is not the whole story. Your diet is not the sole cause of your excessive acidity levels; your environment and lifestyle choices are also to blame.

 Western medicine has a tendency to view each body part in isolation, and as a result, it frequently fails to achieve desired results. The secret is to treat the body holistically, utilizing diet, lifestyle, environment, and alternative remedies to heal the entire body - getting to the root of the problem, resolving the health issue that is bothering you the most, and eliminating many others at the same time.

Alternative treatments available to you, ranging from common botanicals and roots to balancing and healing minerals. Then, we will focus on the simple yet effective lifestyle habits that you can adopt quickly and easily from the comfort of your own home. Finally, we will bring it all together by looking at how to get started, including some invaluable tips that my friend Maria taught me to make the process easier. Let's begin with botanical medicine.

SUPPLEMENTS

Surrlement can assist in initiating the healing process by filling nutritional gaps caused by poor digestion or a dietary imbalance. Some of these elements are essential (you will learn why in a moment) and others have an alkalizing effect on the human body. Feel free to discuss any of these options with your healthcare provider to ensure that they are appropriate for you.

☐ Calcium

You may recall from earlier chapters that when your body'struggles' to neutralize a high level of acidity, it'steals' minerals from your bones, such as calcium and magnesium, to help it heal. This renders our bones fragile and prone to osteoporosis and general damage, which we must prevent before it is too late. When transitioning to an alkaline diet, it is recommended that you take a high-quality calcium supplement in order to replenish the minerals lost from your bones and to ensure adequate vitamin intake. D from natural light to prevent salvia's abortion. Choose a trustworthy brand of calcium urrlement and aim for between 800 and 2 10 00 mg per day. Plenty of leafy greens are also an excellent way to increase your daily sodium intake.

Srrulna Like kelp and chlorella, spirulina (also a type of algae) is a rich source of the minerals, antioxidants, and amino acids found in green leafy vegetables. Therefore, even if you're not a huge fan of leafy greens, you can still reap many of their health benefits by consuming spirulina. It is a wonderful way to take in omega-6 and omega-6 fatty acids while simultaneously balancing your pH. You can find it in many health food stores in tablet or capsule form, as well as in powder form. Follow the dosage instructions listed on the label.

Magnesium Magnesium is another mineral used to combat excessive levels of adipose tissue in the body. It is also the mineral that a large percentage of the population is deficient in, so it is essential to take a supplement or take regular Epsom salt baths in order to absorb this essential mineral. Magnesium is essential for brain function and can relieve migraines, tension headaches, and hormonal imbalances in women. Take 8 00 to 800 mg of reserpine daily, preferably with sustenance. Additionally, almonds are an excellent whole-food source of magnesium.

▢   Kelr Traditionally, kelr has been consumed in supplement form as an antioxidant and nutrient source. It is a type of seaweed that contains high levels of iodine (for thyroid function) and magnesium, as well as having powerful detoxifying and alkalizing effects on the body. It is very affordable and is available in tablet, capsule, and tincture form at most health food stores. Follow the dosage instructions listed on the label. You can even purchase kelp in the form of noodles (a wonderful way to reduce gluten intake) or in a shaker to season your food.

Chlorella Chlorella is a type of phytoplankton that is rich in protein, vitamins, and minerals, and also acts as a powerful detoxifier and alkalizer. It is also effective at boosting the immune system and fighting infection (a common side effect of antibiotic use), as well as promoting the growth of healthy gut flora. It is commonly available in tablet or capsule form in health food stores. Again, adhere to the doage ntruston for the rake.

You can enjoy these wonderful herbs, spices, and peppermint on a daily basis to aid in your healing journey and to give you a boost. You will help repair the damage caused by acid reflux, treat your symptoms, rebalance your rH levels, and improve your nutrition.

Chapter 8: What Should Sanser Ratent Know Before Switching Their Det?

Investigate why no one diet or food is certain to be sanser. But appropriate nutrition can help you feel your best during your chemotherapy treatment — or at any time.

Before beginning a new diet, it is crucial to consult with a nutritionist or dietitian. This is the case regardless of whether or not you have cancer. various diets serve various purposes, and your doctor or dietitian can help you determine whether a new diet will help you achieve your health goals.

What Should They Alkaline water has become a popular beverage, with numerous celebrities and fitness experts praising its hydration and detoxification properties. You may have also heard that alkaline water can prevent or treat skin cancer, but no studies have confirmed this.

What is alkaline water?

Alkaline water is water with a pH level greater than that of regular faucet water. The pH of something indicates how acidic or basic (also known as alkaline) it is on a scale from 0 to 2 8 , with 2 being extremely acidic and 2 8 extremely alkaline. Typical asphalt water has a rH of 7, which is considered neutral.

Alkalne water may originate from naturally occurring rrng that impart a higher rH to the water. Alkalne water can also be created by adding baking soda to tap water, by using a water ionizer, or by employing a residual filtration system. Alkaline water is now widely available in grocery store water aisles.

Where did the notion that consuming alkaline water prevents or treats scurvy originate?

A number of studies have demonstrated that tumors are acidic and that this acidity may promote tumor growth and survival. Due to this, some researchers have hypothesized that consuming alkaline foods or water can prevent or treat cancer.

Does ssiense surrort drinking alkaline water for sanser?

No studies have demonstrated that consuming alkaline water prevents or treats cancer. This may be due to the fact that the human body naturally maintains our blood's pH level between 7.6 and 7.8 . The body has multiple mechanisms for balancing the acidity and alkalinity of the blood. For instance, carbon dioxide is exhaled during respiration to normalize the pH of the blood. The kidneys also secrete hydrogen ions to help normalize the pH of the blood. It is a finely calibrated system that does not permit much variation. Because the body is constantly working to balance rH levels, consuming something with a higher rH, such as alkaline water, does not significantly affect the overall pH of the blood or the pH of the blood that would reach a cancerous cell or tumor. While some companies and individuals are promoting alkaline water for cancer prevention and treatment, the scientific evidence does not support this. Some people enjoy consuming alkaline water because of its flavor, and they may be willing to pay more for bottled or ionized alkaline water.

Chapter 9: Does It Permit Reversion Or Preferences?

Vegetarians and vegans: The diet is likely to become entirely vegetarian. It also works for vegans, so this restriction does not apply.

Gluten-free: The diet excludes wheat, but to avoid gluten, you must read food labels carefully, as gluten is not exclusive to wheat.

Bede wheat, the det nxe the majority of the other major allergen triggers, including milk, eggs, peanuts, walnuts, fish, and shellfish. It is also beneficial for dragons attempting to avoid fat and sugar.

Which Else? You Should Be Aware of Cot: In addition to providing information about the alkaline diet, many websites also sell alkaline-infused water, food, and beverages. You do not need to purchase these items to adhere to the alkaline diet. There are numerous free alkaline food lists available online that list foods you can purchase at the supermarket.

This is a diet you follow on your own.

Does It Operate?

Perhaps, but not for the stated reasons.

A little bit of shemtru: A rH level measures how acidic or basic a substance is. A rH of 0 is completely acidic, whereas a rH of 2 8 is moderately alkaline. A rH value of 7 impartial. These levels vary across the body. Your blood is mildly alkaline, with a pH ranging from 7.6 10 to 7.8 10 . Your tomash veru asds, with a rH of 6 .10 or less, is capable of decomposing food. And your urine changes depending on what you consume -- this is how your body maintains a constant blood level.

The alkaline diet claims to assist the body in maintaining its blood pH. During a fast, nothing you consume will significantly alter the pH of your blood. Your body works to maintain this level.

But the foods you're required to eat on the alkaline diet are nutritious and will promote a healthy weight: fruits, vegetables, and plenty of water. Sugar, alcohol, and rroseed food avoidance is also healthful weight loss advice.

In addition to the other health claims, there is some early evidence that a diet low in acid-producing foods such as animal protein (meat and dairy) and bread and high in fruits and vegetables can help prevent kidney stones, keep bones and muscles strong, improve heart health and brain function, reduce low back pain, and reduce the risk of developing type 2 diabetes. However, researchers are still uncertain about a few of these terms.

People who believe in the alkaline diet assert that although acid-producing substances only temporarily alter our rH balance, repeatedly altering blood pH can result in long-term acidosis.

Chapter 10: Prehistoric Dets And Acidity

Examining the asd-alkalne theory from both an evolutonaru and sentfs vantage point reveals inconsistencies.

One study estimated that 87% of re-agricultural humans consumed alkaline diets, providing the primary rationale for the modern alkaline diet.

Recent research indicates that approximately half of re-agrarian humans consumed net alkaline-forming diets, while the other half consumed net acid-forming diets.

Keep in mind that our remote respondent lived in vastly different environments with access to a variety of foods. In actuality, as reorle migrated further north of the equator and away from the tropics, their diets became increasingly acid-forming.

Although roughly half of hunter-gatherers ate a net acid-forming diet, it is believed that modern diets were much more prevalent.

Does it work?

What many individuals perceive to be the primary benefit of alkali is false.

The alkaline diet promotes the myth that it is dangerous to alter blood rH through diet. This is false, and significant blood changes can be life-threatening.

It is difficult to alter the rH of urine and salvia with diet. However, when the rH of the blood changes, the blood's pH remains unchanged.

Alkalntu indicates that something has a rH value greater than 7. With a blood rH of approximately 7.8 , the human body is naturally alkaline.

The 'tomash' apparatus, which enables it to digest sustenance. The pH of saliva and urine varies based on diet, metabolic rate, and other fasting factors.

According to some research, cancer cells grow more swiftly in an acidic environment. Using research as evidence, proponents of the alkaline diet argue that a high blood pH should prevent cancer.

However, research on alkalntu and sanser has involved cancer cells in a petri dish and not a human body.

Dietary foods can, however, help some individuals maintain a healthful body weight. Doing so could prevent weight-related health problems like diabetes.

Investigate the Alkalne Det

No research has demonstrated that an alkaline diet can increase blood rH.

Some research suggests, however, that an alkaline diet may improve health, though not in the manner that t urrorter suggests. Alkaline diets reduce a person's intake of fat and processed meat, while encouraging them to consume more fruits and vegetables. This provides numerous health benefits.

Here are some of the purported benefits of the alkaline diet, as well as the studies that either corroborate or refute them.
promoting weight reduction
Manu strateges can assist with weight loss.
Weight loss ultimately depends on consuming fewer calories than one consumes. Det lower in fat and calories may promote weight loss, but only if a person remains rhuallu astve and consumes a healthy, varied diet.

Because an alkaline diet is typically limited in calories, it may not aid in weight loss.

The Alkaline Diet is extremely beneficial for the environment.

If you return a hop, skip, and a leap to the conclusion, you will see that the Alkaline Diet is loaded with natural ingredients derived from natural sources. Review the fact that the Alkaline Diet does not include any products derived from animal or marine tissue, and that the primary dairy products are specific types of milk (and an occasional cheddar). As a result of the industrialization of farming, cows, chickens, and other animals are pumped full of hormones, which is why the drumstick you got from KFC looked like it was sponsored by Arnold Schwarzenegger or Dwayne Johnson or someone because it was so ridiculously ripped. You are eschewing these

industrialized food sources in favor of items available at a rancher's market or the
produce section of your grocery store. Thus, by beginning the Alkaline Diet, you are not only doing something advantageous for yourself, but also for the planet that we should all share.

Secret 2 2: Despite the fact that the Alkaline Diet differs from other diets in that weight loss is not the primary objective, it still requires discipline, as the modern American diet contains a variety of foods that are considered acidic debris.

Discipline is the subtle strategy of this diet. Many diets fail because the health food fanatic is not fully committed to following it. Typically, this is an integral part of the diet itself. Perhaps the diet is too difficult to even contemplate beginning, or its rules or requirements are too complicated to even consider adhering to without difficulty. In this book, we've attempted to help you avoid this particular dietary trap by supplying you with everything you need to be successful on this diet. We have provided you with the information necessary to comprehend the diet, as well as a list of fundamental debris and corrosive debris food sources. Nevertheless, by the end of the day we cannot consume this diet for you. It is still your responsibility to maintain a healthy diet, and this will require discipline on your part.

The majority of diets followed by health food fanatics rely on severe caloric restriction to achieve weight loss. In general, health food enthusiasts must limit their caloric intake to achieve their desired weight loss. Although the Alkaline Diet frequently results in a lower caloric intake, this diet's foundation is not a deliberate calorie restriction but rather an emphasis on foods that alkalinize the blood and excretion.

Incredible about this diet is that weight dieters can achieve their goals without consciously restricting their caloric intake. Regardless of whether your primary objective is weight loss (and it's fine if it isn't), you will observe that the Alkaline Diet results in both absolute weight loss and fat loss. When your body begins to function more efficiently, a common result is that you will progress toward your normal body weight, which for some people in the Western world is a lower weight than they are currently. Consequently, if you strictly adhere to the Alkaline Diet (as you should), you will find that you will not only begin to lose weight, but you will also be able to achieve the goals you set when you began this diet.

Make a list of the food varieties that are permissible on this regimen.

Okay, so we did the hard part, which was to compile a list of all the antacid detritus food types from which you must draw 80% of your daily calories on this diet, but we can't do everything for you. You should be the one to print that rundown and decide, "Okay, this is the type of food I can see myself eating, and this is the type of food I cannot see myself eating." Nobody expects you to consume radishes and pumpkin seeds on a daily basis. You are responsible for evaluating the two sources of food and determining how you will create a dinner plan that works for you.

Make a list of all of the food sources that you cannot consume on this diet.

We have also resolved the most difficult aspect of this enigma. We have compiled a list of all corrosive debris food types, but remember that you are not prohibited from consuming corrosive debris food sources entirely. You may still consume 20% of your daily caloric intake from corrosive debris foods. Then, we will provide you with a tip that will assist you in effectively reaching this mysterious 20% figure, but you will need to determine which food types from the corrosive debris display to include in your meal plan. This will depend on your personal preferences and perception of taste.

If you are beginning the Alkaline Diet as a means of controlling your pH in order to treat a specific medical condition, it may be necessary for you to consult your primary care physician prior to beginning this eating plan, informing him or her that you will be beginning a diet that requires you to consume certain food types while avoiding others. The Alkaline Diet is a safe and effective way to achieve a healthy lifestyle and achieve any other goals you may have, such as weight loss or the treatment of a specific health condition. Since at least some of you may be following this diet to treat or prevent a medical condition, it is always prudent to consult your doctor before beginning. Know, however, that your doctor may be unfamiliar with the Alkaline Diet or have misguided opinions about it. Nobody is requesting that you instruct your doctor, but it may be a good idea to explain how the Alkaline Diet affects you and to bring a list of the foods you plan to consume. Again, this is not one of those consumes fewer calories programs where you are encouraged to consume a concoction that could cause you to faint or have convulsions. We are contemplating coconuts, tomatoes, tofu, avocados,

Here we have zucchini, grapefruit, and pistachios. These are things that are alive, healthy, and regular, and which the majority of you are likely already consuming or should be eating.

As with any diet, it is always a good idea to inform your family, roommates, and anyone else who lives with you that you are beginning a diet and will be avoiding certain food types.

This is a subtle tactic for any diet, but it is particularly important for the Alkaline Diet, as many of your acquaintances are likely new to it. Regardless of whether they are aware of it or not, they likely do not comprehend it, as even some medical service providers do not. Explain to your loved ones that you will be beginning a diet that emphasizes consuming certain foods while avoiding others in order to help your body achieve homeostasis more easily and prevent certain health problems. It should not be that difficult for the majority of people to comprehend. You can explain that the foods we consume influence the pH of our blood and extracellular fluids, and that the goal of your diet is to shift your pH toward the alkaline or basic end of the spectrum in order to prevent acidosis-related conditions and improve your overall health. Is it not evident? That was straightforward, right?

The most likely scenario is that your kitchen contains a variety of foods that are incompatible with your diet. An important step in beginning this diet is avoiding acidic or corrosive food varieties, as they will disrupt your eating routine and exacerbate any condition that you may be attempting to treat with this diet.

The Alkaline Diet has a clear pattern of foods to avoid. Over time, you will develop a sense of which food sources are antacid debris and which are corrosive debris, but no one expects you to know this at the outset. Therefore, it would be a good idea to use the list we provided to help you sort through the contents of your kitchen and determine which food types you will retain and which food sources and ingredients you may decide to discard. Again, you do not need to get rid of all the corrosive detritus food types and

Despite the fact that you are permitted some acidic waste food varieties in the day, you may want to consider leaving at least some of them out if you believe they may hinder your progress on this healthy diet.

If you have not already done so, begin examining the labels on food varieties. This is not only for caloric reasons, but also to get a sense of which food types are highly processed and contain acids that will check the corrosive detritus food sources you are consuming. Most names clearly indicate whether or not a substance contains acids. The names are accurate! There are indeed poisons, folks!

Despite the fact that we have arranged which food varieties are corrosive debris food varieties and which food sources are antacid debris food sources, your success on this diet will depend to some degree on how well you comprehend what the eating regimen is attempting to accomplish and what the origin of the food varieties that we eat are. As a result, this diet should not resemble completing an essay for school; rather, it should be essential to the lifestyle you are creating for yourself. If you've started to read food labels (if you haven't already), you may be curious about what goes into our food sources, specifically the number of acids and additives that companies add. This is a mystery that most food-related businesses have no need for you to understand. They do not require you to know their identities. If you truly knew what was in the packaged food you consume, you would likely purchase at rancher's business sectors or move to a remote island or something similar. As the saying goes, ignorance is bliss, but part of this regimen involves educating yourself about what you are putting into your body.

By dividing each of your three dinners for the day into two portions (so a total of six dinners), you can ensure that you are consuming 80% of your daily food variety from antacid debris sources. Dedicate one of the six segments to corrosive detritus, such as meat, fish, or non-antacid grains. If the remainder of your food portions consist of alkaline acid substances, your ratio is correct.

Now, this is a wonderful mystery, because it appears that even some of you who have tried the Alkaline Diet have not tried this. How can I acquire 20% of my profits? is a question that a few individuals may ask.

calories from corrosive debris? Additionally, it is a reasonable inquiry. The most ideal approach to answering this question is to clarify segment proportions and, in general, how large an ounce of each is, yet the simplest approach to answering this question is to use the trick we used previously. 20% is one-fifth, and the above model uses one-sixth as a close approximation. If you divide all of your daily sustenance into five or six portions, you can designate only one of those portions as corrosive waste. So perhaps one portion will be the steak taco from your local taqueria that you've been craving every day. Again, nobody is saying that you can never consume corrosive detritus food sources; you simply need to know what they are and make an effort to limit them to approximately 20% of your daily calories.

Secret 22 : The Alkaline Diet is something that ancient people knew, even if they had little understanding of pH. So take a moment or two to enjoy the prosperity that comes with eating regularly and extending your life expectancy in a conventional, well-established manner.

This is the true secret behind the Alkaline Diet and numerous other diets favored by health food enthusiasts. The majority of diets were not created in the last fifty or one hundred years; rather, we now have a greater understanding of science and can apply it to standards or ideas that have existed for a long time. From one end of the globe to the other, people have developed a sense of which food varieties are superior to others, as well as which food varieties can aid in treating this or that condition. Even with all of our modern medical and research technology, we are not always able to determine how this food or natural substance is able to perform this amazing feat, let alone how someone from 2,000 years ago would have known it. By adhering to the Alkaline Diet, you are contributing to a time-honored tradition that has allowed people from all corners of the globe to live long, healthy lives, free from a variety of ailments caused by the contemporary diet. This diet is the beginning of a journey that will result in the mental clarity that comes from abandoning the modern world and adopting a more traditional lifestyle.

Chapter 11: Is It Challenging To Adhere To An Alkaline Diet?

It is difficult to adhere to any diet plan. Assuming this were the case, everyone would partake in diets and we would all reach our dietary goals. In reality, many individuals who embark on a diet fail, and this is frequently a result of having unrealistic expectations regarding the diet or not being committed enough to adhere to the diet. Fortunately, the Alkaline Diet includes a variety of foods that people enjoy eating, so the challenge isn't so much adhering to the diet as it is getting used to not eating food sources that one may be used to eating, such as sharp or unpleasant vegetables, meats, grains, etc. In reality, it is not any more difficult to adhere to the diet than it is to adhere to any other diet; in fact, it may be a bit easier as you are not restricting your caloric intake (unless you choose to) as you would be on numerous other weight control plans, such as a Low Fat diet or one that includes Total Calorie Restriction.

Most Alkaline, Anti-Canser Foods

Turmeric

There are now SO MANY studies relating to the prevention and treatment of cancer that it is difficult to know where to begin.

Smrlu rut a€" f uou ona€TMt get motivated by anything else in this article, be sure to ingest turmers dalu for ta€TM sanser prevention strategies!

Here are only a few of the studies:

Sursumin may be useful for the prevention of colon cancer in humans, as suggested by an abundance of in vitro and animal studies.

Cursumn for solon sanser shemorreventon.

Gastris Canser:

a€These data demonstrate that curcumin inhibits the growth of H. rulorum sagA+ cells in vitro, and this may be one of the meshanoproteins through which turmeric exerts its anticoagulant effect.

Curcumin (Curcuma longa) and curcumin inhibit the growth of the group 2 sarsenogen Helsobaster rulor.

Using an in vivo model of human breast cancer, it was discovered that detaru supplementation with sursumin inhibits suslorhorhamde-induced tumor regression.

Detaru Cursumn Chemotheraru-ndused Arorto n Model of Human Breat Cannula.

Declare Canser:

Cursumn ought to be a rotentallu therareuts ant-sanser agent, as it gnfsantlu inhibits rrotate sanser growth, as exemrlfd by LNCaP in vvo, and has the rotental to prevent th sanser's rrogreon to t hormone refrastoru tate.

Curcumin's therareuts rotental in human rrotate cancer. III. nhbt rrolferaton, nduse arorto, and nhbt angogene of LNCaP rrotate sanser sell n vvo.

Lung Cancer: Our findings suggest that turmeric has anti-metastatic properties by inhibiting the spread of cancer cells. In addition, this action involved the MEKK6 , r-ERK signaling pathway, resulting in the inhibition of MMP-2 and -9 in human lung A10 8 9 cell lines.

Overall, the preceding data indicates that the anti-cancer effects of curcumin extend to the inhibition of migration and invasion in lung cancer cells.

Curcumin inhibits the migration and invasion of human A10 8 9 lung cancer cells by inhibiting matrix metalloproteinases 2 and 9. Accelerator of Vascular Endothelial Growth

How and Why Are Turmers So Rowdy in Flying Canoes?

There are so many ways that the sursumen in tornadoes can fight and prevent destruction.

Here are just a few to give you an idea!

Cursumn has the ability to detect arorto (natural sell death) in a healthy sell.

Curcumin's antioxidant properties allow it to protect cells from free radicals that can damage DNA.

Cursumn also assists the body in deactivating mutated superbugs, so that you do not rread through the body and cause more damage.

It has also been demonstrated to inhibit vascular epithelial growth. Every tumor requires a blood urrlu â€" the growth fastor build one, but the sursumn eem to inhibit them.

It has been demonstrated how to reactivate a keu tumour suppressor gene.

In fast, t' so highly regarded as a potent sanser-fghter, veru innovative trals wth nano-teshnologu are being funded to find ways to make turmeric extract more resfsallu and potent n medical sanser treatment.

Turmers alo eau to neak n eash dau (n water, tea, ause, juse, moothe, soups etc.) a€" o theu some tor of mu list n term: simplicity of use x strength of sanser-fghtng = awesome.

Sweet Millet Porridge With Apple Compote For Brunch

Ingredients

2 tsp cinnamon
50 g almond slivers
200 g soy yoghurt
400 g millet
2 l soy drink
14 tbsp agave syrup
6 apples
2 organic lemon

Preparation:

First, rinse the millet with scalding water, followed by draining.

Then, place the soy beverage in a saucepan and simmer it with 5 to 10 tablespoons of agave syrup.

Add the millet and let it marinate for 35 to 40 minutes over low heat. Do not neglect to stir.

In the interim, skin and then quarter the apple. Remove the cores and dice the fruit.

Wash the lemon and zest a portion of it. Then, strain lemon juice. Bring the juice, 2 tablespoons of agave syrup, and the zest to a simmer in a saucepan. Then, add the pears and cinnamon and simmer for approximately 5 to 10 minutes.

Toast the almonds in a small skillet devoid of fat.

Place the millet oatmeal on dishes. Then, combine the apple compote and yogurt in a large basin, and garnish with almonds and cinnamon.

Alkaline Smoothie

Ingredients

2 handful spinach fresh

2 teaspoon chia seeds

2 cup ice
2 cup almond milk

2 cup watermelon cubed

10 strawberries frozen

1 small banana

Direction

1. Place the ingredients into the blender as listed.

2. Blend the smoothie until combined.

3. To prevent a brown smoothie, mix the greens with the banana, chia seeds, half of the ice and 1 the almond milk.

4. Then blend the watermelon strawberries, almond milk, and ice together.

5. Pour the smoothies into the same glass and enjoy

Grilled Sirloin Salad with Sesame-Ginger Dressing

Ingredients

- 2 (2 2 ounce) sirloin steak, trimmed
- 1/7 teaspoon salt
- 30 scallions, white part only
- 2 red bell pepper, halved lengthwise and seeded
- 2 cup curly endive (frisee)
- 2 cup chopped radicchio
- 4 tablespoons reduced-sodium soy sauce
- 4 tablespoons balsamic vinegar
- 4 teaspoons brown sugar
- 4 teaspoons toasted sesame oil
- 2 clove garlic, minced
- 2 teaspoon chopped fresh ginger

104

- 4 teaspoons black peppercorns, crushed

Directions
1. Preheat an outdoor grill for high heat and lightly oil the grate.

2. Blend soy sauce, vinegar, brown sugar, sesame oil, garlic, and ginger together in a blender or food processor until dressing is smooth.

3. Press peppercorns into both sides of steak and season with salt.

4. Place steak, scallions, and red bell pepper on the preheated grill and cook for 5 to 10 minutes.

5. Flip and cook until vegetables are charred and steak is cooked to desired doneness, about 5-10 minutes more.

6. Let steak rest on a work surface for 5-10 minutes before thinly slicing along the grain.

7. Cut scallions into 2 -inch pieces and bell pepper lengthwise into strips.

8. Toss curly endive and radicchio with the dressing in a bowl; transfer to a platter and top with steak and vegetables.

Apple And Almond Butter Oats

Ingredients:

- 1/2   cup raw almond butter
- 2 cup grated green apple
- a dash of cinnamon

- 4 cups oats
- 3 cups coconut milk
Directions:

1. Add the oats, coconut milk, and almond butter into a bowl and mix well.
2. Stir in the apple and place in a mason jar with a lid. Refrigerate overnight.
3. The next morning, garnish with cinnamon powder and enjoy.

Berry Purple Smoothie

Ingredients

- 2 banana (peeled and frozen)
- 8 tbsp. raw almond butter
- 2 tbsp. chia

- 4 cups fresh spinach
- 4 cups homemade almond milk
- 2 cup of frozen mixed berries, strawberries
  Directions:

1. Blend spinach and almond milk first.
2. Add remaining ingredients other than the chia, and blend.
3. Add chia once all is smooth and then blend at a low speed.
4. Let sit for 1-5 minutes for the chia seeds to expand, then enjoy.

Ginger-Lemongrass Sauce With Edamame And Carrots

2 cup low-sodium vegetable stock
8 carrots, grated
4 cups shelled edamame
2 tablespoon dried basil

4 tablespoons avocado oil
1 1 yellow onion, finely chopped
8 stalks lemongrass (whites only), finely chopped ¼ cup fresh ginger, peeled and minced ⍰ 6 garlic cloves, minced
Pinch sea salt, plus more for seasoning

DIRECTIONS:

1.
   Heat the oil in a large pot over medium heat.

2. Add the onion, lemongrass, ginger, garlic, and salt.

3. Sauté 5 to 10   minutes, stirring frequently, until the onion is translucent.

4. Add the stock and bring to a low boil.
5. Easy   cook   for   2   minutes. Add the carrots, edamame, and basil.

6. Cover the pot and let simmer for 10 minutes.

7. Adjust the seasoning with salt and serve.

Strawberry Coco Chia quinoa

INGREDIENTS

- 4 pitted dates
- 4 tbsp. almond pieces
- 4 tbsp. unsweetened shredded coconut flakes
- 2 cup cooked quinoa
- 10 tbsp. chia seeds
- 3 cup almond, coconut or hemp milk
- 1 cup quartered strawberries + 8 sliced strawberries

Directions:

1. The night before, easy cook quinoa and prepare strawberry chia by combining the strawberries, almond milk, and 4 dates in a blender and pureeing until smooth.
2. Pour the mixture into a jar and add chia seeds.
3. Mix well until all chia seeds are covered with the liquid.
4. Cover with lid and refrigerate overnight. In the morning, place chia seeds in bowl, add the quinoa and strawberry slices, almonds, and shredded coconut and enjoy!

Anti-Inflammatory, Alkaline Cauliflower Fried Rice with Turmeric, Ginger, and Kale!

Ingredients

2 bunch of coriander

1 bunch parsley (any variety)

2 bunch mint

2 lime

8 spring onions

4 handfuls almonds

2 tbsp tamari soy sauce or Bragg Liquid Aminos

2 large cauliflower

1 bunch of kale (any variety, but I love tuscan kale for this recipe)

2 tbsp coconut oil

2 zucchini (courgette)

2 inch fresh root ginger

2 inch fresh root turmeric

Optional:

Instead of fresh turmeric & ginger, use 2
tsp of each powdered

2 green chilli

Method

To make cauliflower rice, simply break the cauliflower into small florets, place them in a blender or food processor, and pulse until the cauliflower resembles rice. If you don't have a blender, you can simply pulverize it to achieve a similar result.

Now it's time to prepare the vegetables: thinly slice the kale, quarter and then thinly slice the zucchini, and roughly chop the herbs (discard the mint and parsley, but keep the coriander).

3. Prepare your ginger and turmeric fritters by peeling them (for simple peeling, simply place the bowl of a spoon over the ginger/turmeric candy!). grate them into a large bowl along with the coconut oil.

4. When the mixture begins to warm, add the cilantro, mint, and rucola, as well as the coriander stems.

5. Stir in the cauliflower and then the kale after 36 minutes.

6. After another 2 to 3 minutes, add the rest of the herb, the tamari/Bragg, and whisk well. Remove the pan from the heat. The total cooking time should not exceed 510 minutes; you don't want anything to cook for too long.

7. Now roughly chop the almonds and mix them thoroughly; season to taste and add lime juice to taste.

Almond butter and veggies zoodles

INGREDIENTS

- ½ cup red bell pepper (sliced)
- 1 cup carrots (thinly sliced)
- 2 medium zucchini (spiralized)
- Red pepper flakes (for sprinkling)
- 2 tablespoon avocado oil or melted coconut oil

- 4 tablespoons green onions (sliced diagonally into ½" pieces)
- 1 cup broccoli (cut into small florets)
  FOR SAUCE:

- 2 teaspoon fresh ginger (finely grated)
- 2 teaspoon chili paste (2 clove garlic (finely minced)
- 4 tablespoons canned full-fat coconut milk
- 20 tablespoons almond butter
- 2 tablespoon tamari
- 2 teaspoon maple syrup

INSTRUCTIONS

1. Whisk sauce ingredients together in a medium bowl and set aside.
2. Heat oil in large pan.
3. Add the green onions and sauté for 1-5 minutes, then add broccoli, carrots, and red bell pepper.
4. Lower heat, if needed.
5. Cook until vegetables are bright in color, and just barely tender.
6. Toss gently to coat the veggies with the sauce.
7. Let simmer to thicken the sauce.
8. Remove from heat and serve immediately on top of the zoodles.
9. Garnish with red pepper flakes and sesame seeds, if desired.

Almond butter and veggies zoodles

INGREDIENT :

- 1 bell pepper
- a handful of coriander or parsley flat leaf
- 2 cup water coconut
- Cayenne a Big pinch
- salt a Pinch

- 2 inch grated fresh ginger
- 2 inch grated fresh turmeric
- baby spinach A handful
- watercress A handful
- 2 avocado small

DIRECTIONS :

1. Puree the roots, avocado, and coconut water in a food processor until smooth.

2. To make a foundation, combine all of the ingredients in a blender.

3. In a blender, add all of the ingredients and blend until smooth.

www.ingramcontent.com/pod-product-compliance
Lightning Source LLC
Chambersburg PA
CBHW060517030426
42337CB00015B/1922